THE ULTIMATE DYSPHAGIA DIET COOKBOOK

Deliciously Simple Recipes Tailored For Every Phase of the Dysphagia Diet Levels (Pureed, Mechanical Soft, Advanced Soft, and Regular Stages)

Michael Slowick, RDN

COPYRIGHT PAGE

for a particular purpose. While every effort has been made to ensure the accuracy of the information provided herein, no promises are made regarding its completeness or accuracy. Any statements made by sales employees or representatives, whether verbal or written, do not constitute extended or implied guarantees.

Table of Contents

INTRODUCTION

Dysphagia is the term used to describe the struggle with swallowing, and it can stem from various sources like nerve or muscle issues or blockages in the throat or esophagus. Figuring out what's causing it and finding ways to manage it is crucial for staying healthy and avoiding problems like malnutrition, dehydration, or feeling isolated.

When you have dysphagia, swallowing isn't as smooth as it should be. It's like there's a glitch in the system—your muscles and nerves aren't quite working together right, so swallowing can feel awkward or sluggish. Sometimes, you might even cough or choke when trying to swallow liquids, food, or your own spit.

A lot of people have had moments where they've felt like something went down the wrong way or like there's a lump in their throat after eating too quickly. That's kind of what dysphagia feels like, though usually it's nothing to worry about. However, if it sticks around, especially after a stroke, it might be a sign of something more serious. If dysphagia isn't treated, it can lead to complications like food going into your airway, which can cause lung infections or pneumonia.

A specialist called a speech-language pathologist (SLP) can check out your swallowing ability and offer treatments if needed. Dysphagia can affect anyone, but it's more common in older folks. Treatments vary depending on what's causing the swallowing issues.

CHAPTER I: THE SIGNIFICANCE OF DEALING WITH DYSPHAGIA

The term dysphagia, originating from the Greek words "dys," denoting "difficulty," and "phago," indicating "to eat," serves as a descriptor for a condition that transcends mere inconvenience, delving into the intricate mechanics of swallowing. Dysphagia, at its essence, serves as a descriptor for instances where swallowing becomes arduous or painful. Despite the apparent simplicity of swallowing, it entails a sophisticated coordination of numerous muscles and nerves operating in synchrony.

The complexity of dysphagia becomes evident upon contemplation of its ramifications on an individual's overall health, happiness, and quality of life. It extends beyond mere physical discomfort and may precipitate additional challenges such as malnutrition, dehydration, and an elevated susceptibility to aspiration pneumonia. Essentially, dysphagia manifests as a symptom indicative of disruption within the intricate network of muscles and nerves indispensable for swallowing, resulting in difficulties in ingesting food or liquids.

A myriad of anatomical and neurological factors can contribute to the onset of this disorder, encompassing conditions ranging from tumors to gastroesophageal reflux disease (GERD). To devise personalized approaches for dysphagia diagnosis, treatment, and management, a thorough exploration of the disorder's etiology and multifaceted manifestations is imperative.

Dysphagia is conceptualized in a manner that reflects a nuanced understanding of the condition, one that encompasses not only the mechanics of swallowing but also its broader implications for an individual's well-being and quality of life. This comprehension serves as the foundation for a compassionate and comprehensive strategy aimed at addressing dysphagia, fostering an environment where individuals grappling with this issue can access the support and assistance they need.

The significance of managing dysphagia

A comprehensive comprehension of the extensive implications of dysphagia on an individual's health and overall quality of life necessitates a recognition of the imperative nature of resolving this disorder. Dysphagia, characterized by challenges or discomfort in swallowing, presents a multifaceted issue that demands attention and diligent management; it transcends being a mere inconvenience during meal times. Despite its seemingly innocuous nature, swallowing is, in fact, a highly intricate neurological and muscular process that requires precise synchronization. Any disruption to this intricate process, as seen in dysphagia, yields repercussions that extend far beyond the dining experience.

The peril of malnutrition and dehydration looms large when dysphagia remains unaddressed or poorly managed. Difficulties in swallowing often prompt individuals to reduce their food and water intake, leaving their bodies deprived of essential nutrients and hydration. Resulting consequences may include diminished energy levels, compromised health, and prolonged recovery periods due to nutritional imbalances.

Moreover, dysphagia heightens the risk of aspiration pneumonia—a severe condition where food, liquids, or saliva enter the airway instead of the digestive tract. Aspiration pneumonia poses a significant threat to respiratory health, precipitating respiratory infections and complications. Hence, addressing dysphagia serves as a proactive measure against such adverse outcomes, not only safeguarding physical health but also alleviating emotional and psychological burdens associated with chronic health conditions.

Furthermore, dysphagia can exert a profound impact on an individual's mental and social well-being. The challenges and embarrassment associated with navigating meal times amidst swallowing difficulties can lead to social isolation and a decline in overall quality of life. Adopting a holistic approach to dysphagia treatment entails addressing not only the physical symptoms but also attending to the patient's mental, emotional, and social needs.

Given the diverse array of ways in which dysphagia can affect an individual's health and well-being, it is imperative to proactively address this condition. Healthcare professionals, caregivers, and patients alike play pivotal roles in mitigating the adverse effects of dysphagia, enhancing nutritional outcomes, and bolstering quality of life by fostering awareness of the condition and implementing effective management strategies.

CHAPTER II: GRASPING THE PROCESS OF SWALLOWING

Despite its deceptively simple appearance, swallowing is actually a highly intricate physiological process crucial for our survival. To fully grasp the challenges posed by disorders like dysphagia, which disrupt such a complex system, it's imperative to delve into the mechanics of swallowing. This process mirrors a symphony, where each component, from muscles to nerves, plays a vital role in orchestrating a seamless and efficient performance.

Commencing with the oral phase, the intricate interplay of anatomy and physiology comes into play. Here, the tongue, aided by saliva, initiates the breakdown of food into a more digestible consistency. Transitioning to the pharyngeal phase, the chewed bolus is propelled to the rear of the mouth. During this phase, the epiglottis safeguards the airway by preventing food or liquids from entering the trachea while the larynx elevates. Concurrently, the upper esophageal sphincter relaxes, allowing the bolus to commence its journey down the esophagus and into the gastric phase.

The esophageal phase is characterized by peristalsis, a rhythmic muscle contraction resembling a wave, which propels the bolus down the esophagus and into the stomach. The precision required for optimal swallowing is underscored by the seamless and rapid execution of these processes, typically spanning mere seconds.

Dysphagia can stem from a multitude of sources that disrupt this intricate process. Individuals with neurological disorders, anatomical anomalies, or muscle impairments may experience difficulty swallowing due to impaired coordination. Healthcare practitioners must possess a comprehensive understanding of the swallowing mechanism to identify the underlying causes of dysphagia and implement appropriate interventions.

Dysphagia management transcends mere observation of outward symptoms as our understanding of swallowing intricacies deepens. A holistic approach to diagnosis, treatment, and management hinges upon a thorough comprehension of the underlying physiological mechanisms. By comprehending the complexities of this orchestrated movement symphony and addressing the issues dysphagia presents, healthcare providers and individuals can collaborate to enhance the well-being of those affected by dysphagia.

The study of the structure and function of the swallowing process

Swallowing, despite its seemingly effortless nature, is a remarkably intricate physiological process crucial for our survival. To grasp the challenges posed by disorders like dysphagia, which disrupt such a complex system, delving into the mechanics of swallowing becomes imperative. Similar to a symphony, swallowing entails a harmonious collaboration of various components, encompassing muscles, nerves, and anatomical structures, all essential for achieving a seamless and efficient performance.

The orchestrated sequence of swallowing commences with the oral phase, where anatomy and physiology converge. Here, the tongue, aided by saliva, initiates the breakdown of food into a more digestible consistency. Progressing to the pharyngeal phase, the chewed bolus is propelled to the back of the mouth. During this phase, the epiglottis safeguards the airway by preventing food or liquids from entering the trachea, while the larynx elevates. Simultaneously, the upper esophageal sphincter relaxes, allowing the bolus to commence its descent down the esophagus and into the gastric phase.

Peristalsis, characterized by rhythmic muscular contractions resembling waves, propels the bolus through the esophagus and into the stomach during the esophageal phase. The precision demanded for optimal swallowing is underscored by the seamless and rapid execution of these processes, typically taking only a few seconds.

Dysphagia can arise from various factors that disrupt this intricate process. Individuals with neurological disorders, anatomical anomalies, or muscle impairments may experience difficulty swallowing due to a lack of coordination required for the process. Healthcare practitioners must possess a comprehensive understanding of the swallowing mechanism to identify the underlying etiologies of dysphagia and administer appropriate interventions.

The management of dysphagia necessitates more than mere surface-level observation as we delve deeper into the nuances of swallowing. A holistic approach to diagnosis, treatment, and management is facilitated by a thorough comprehension of the underlying physiological mechanisms. Collaboratively, healthcare providers and individuals can enhance the well-being of those grappling with dysphagia by comprehending the intricacies of this orchestrated movement symphony and devising strategies to address the challenges it presents.

Phases of the Swallowing Process

The act of sucking entails a remarkably intricate process, involving a series of interdependent steps meticulously orchestrated to transport food and liquids from the oral cavity to the stomach in a harmonized manner. This elaborate choreography not only provides insight into the complexity of swallowing but also serves as a critical diagnostic and therapeutic tool in addressing conditions such as dysphagia, which arises when this intricate ballet is disrupted.

Commencing with the oral phase, the initial step of swallowing entails the manipulation and mastication of food by the tongue, accompanied by the incorporation of saliva to facilitate digestion. This phase plays a pivotal role in the formation of a cohesive bolus, the amalgamated mass of chewed food primed for propulsion into subsequent phases of swallowing.

Transitioning to the pharyngeal phase, the bolus is propelled towards the posterior region of the mouth, triggering a cascade of protective mechanisms to safeguard the airway. The epiglottis, akin to a flap, descends to shield the airway, while the larynx elevates to seal off the trachea, ensuring that the bolus traverses the esophagus rather than the windpipe, thereby averting aspiration. Simultaneously, relaxation of the upper esophageal sphincter facilitates entry of the bolus into the esophagus.

In the esophageal phase, the bolus embarks on its journey downhill towards the stomach, propelled by the rhythmic contractions of esophageal muscles in a process known as peristalsis. This coordinated muscular action facilitates swift and seamless transit of the bolus through the esophagus, culminating in its arrival in the stomach for subsequent digestion.

The orchestration of these multifaceted steps occurs seamlessly and swiftly, typically within the blink of an eye. However, disruptions to any facet of this intricate process can precipitate dysphagia, characterized by difficulty in swallowing. Neurological disorders, anatomical anomalies, or muscular impairments are among the myriad factors that may impede the smooth progression of swallowing, underscoring the importance of a comprehensive understanding of the swallowing process for accurate diagnosis and effective treatment of dysphagia.

In essence, the act of swallowing mirrors a symphony of synchronized movements and precision, emblematic of the remarkable efficiency of the human body. Individuals grappling with dysphagia necessitate tailored interventions aimed at restoring the fluidity of this vital physiological function. However, such interventions can only be rendered efficacious if healthcare practitioners possess a profound appreciation for each stage of swallowing and are equipped to address any impediments encountered along the way.

CHAPTER III: CAUSES, VARIETIES, IDENTIFICATION, AND MANAGEMENT OF DYSPHAGIA

The intricate nature of dysphagia, characterized by impairment in the swallowing process, stems from a myriad of contributing factors spanning neurological, structural, and muscular domains. Neurological disorders such as multiple sclerosis, stroke, Parkinson's disease, and Parkinson's intricately disrupt the cerebral regulatory systems essential for coordinated swallowing. Post-stroke dysphagia, for instance, underscores the critical importance of maintaining optimal neurological health, as damage to the brain's swallowing centers can lead to swallowing difficulties.

Moreover, neurodegenerative conditions like Parkinson's disease can further compound swallowing challenges by affecting the nerves and muscles involved in the process. The inflammatory demyelinating condition multiple sclerosis introduces disruptions to neurological circuits, exacerbating difficulties in swallowing coordination.

Structural causes of dysphagia introduce physical impediments to the smooth passage of food, exemplified by tumors in the throat or esophagus, whether benign or malignant. Gastroesophageal reflux disease (GERD), characterized by acid reflux, underscores the intricate relationship between gastrointestinal health and swallowing function. Over time, GERD-induced esophageal inflammation and scarring can culminate in dysphagia development.

Muscular disorders such as myasthenia gravis and muscular dystrophy further compound swallowing challenges by affecting the muscles responsible for orchestrating swallowing motions. The progressive deterioration characteristic of muscular dystrophy can compromise the integrity of muscles essential for swallowing, mirroring the swallowing dysfunction observed in myasthenia gravis due to muscle weakness induced by inflammation.

Clinical diagnosis of dysphagia relies on discerning the severity and nature of swallowing difficulties, informing tailored treatment approaches. Various levels of dysphagia intervention, from blending meals to facilitate swallowing in severe cases (Level 1) to accommodating softer textures in mild dysphagia (Level 2), highlight the necessity for personalized management strategies.

Comprehensive comprehension of dysphagia is imperative due to its multifaceted etiology, necessitating nuanced and individualized treatment approaches. By discerning the diverse neurological, anatomical, and muscular underpinnings of dysphagia, clinicians can direct targeted interventions to restore swallowing function and enhance the quality of life for individuals grappling with this condition.

Indications and Manifestations of Dysphagia

Individuals grappling with dysphagia, a condition marked by discomfort or difficulty in swallowing, present an array of symptoms and cues that collectively paint a comprehensive picture of the challenges they encounter when endeavoring to transport food and beverages from their mouths to their stomachs. These symptoms encompass various physical manifestations that offer insights into the broader implications of the condition on overall health.

Primarily, dysphagia manifests as impaired swallowing function. Meal times may elongate as individuals struggle to propel food down their esophagus, leading to feelings of frustration when they perceive food to be lodged in their throat or chest. Consequently, alterations in eating habits may arise, with individuals opting for softer-textured meals that require less effort to chew. A common symptom is dysphagia-related coughing or choking episodes, occurring when food or liquid inadvertently enters the airway instead of the esophagus during swallowing.

Due to inadequate food intake resulting from dysphagia-related challenges, individuals may experience unexplained weight loss, highlighting the nutritional deficiencies and dehydration that can ensue as the condition progresses, further compromising overall well-being. Additionally, regurgitation emerges as a prominent symptom, characterized by the regurgitation of partially digested food into the mouth post-swallowing, typically indicative of underlying issues with the lower esophageal sphincter or other components of the swallowing mechanism.

Beyond these overt physical manifestations, dysphagia can also exert social and emotional ramifications. The prospect of encountering difficulties during meals may evoke feelings of anxiety or distress, potentially leading to social withdrawal and a diminished quality of life stemming from a sense of shame or discomfort associated with eating in public settings.

Recognizing and understanding the diverse array of symptoms and indicators associated with dysphagia is imperative for prompt diagnosis and intervention. Beyond merely identifying physical challenges, a comprehensive evaluation must encompass an appreciation of the psychological and social ramifications of the condition. Healthcare providers aim to address dysphagia in a manner that not only restores swallowing function but also enhances overall quality of life for affected individuals. Through diligent recognition and management of these multifaceted signs, healthcare professionals strive to achieve this overarching goal.

CHAPTER IV: DIAGNOSIS OF DYSPHAGIA

The diagnosis of dysphagia is a comprehensive endeavor best undertaken through a collaborative effort by a multi-disciplinary team, integrating clinical evaluations, specialized imaging examinations, and various diagnostic tools to comprehensively assess the nature and scope of swallowing difficulties. Given the intricate nature of dysphagia, a meticulous evaluation is imperative to guide targeted interventions and ensure effective management.

Initiating the diagnostic process involves a meticulous clinical evaluation, encompassing a detailed review of the patient's medical history. Healthcare professionals delve into the onset and progression of symptoms, concurrent medical conditions, and relevant medications. Additionally, a thorough physical examination evaluates oral and pharyngeal health, assessing reflexes, muscular strength, and the coordination of swallowing.

Specialized imaging studies play a pivotal role in enhancing diagnostic precision. The Videofluoroscopic Swallow Study (VFSS) employs dynamic radiography, capturing real-time images of swallowing by administering contrast material with food or beverages. This allows clinicians to observe swallowing dynamics, facilitating early identification of abnormalities. Similarly, the Fiberoptic Endoscopic Evaluation of Swallowing (FEES) involves direct visualization of the pharynx using a flexible endoscope inserted through the nasal passages, providing crucial insights into swallowing anatomy and function.

Supplementary diagnostic modalities, such as pH monitoring for acid reflux and manometry for esophageal pressure assessment, may also be employed to elucidate underlying pathophysiology. Furthermore, monitoring nutritional status through blood tests becomes pertinent in cases of significant weight loss. Occasionally, advanced imaging techniques like CT scans or MRIs are utilized to detect structural abnormalities or tumors contributing to dysphagia.

Collaboration among healthcare providers is paramount throughout the diagnostic process. Consultation with specialists including neurologists, gastroenterologists, and speech-language pathologists ensures a comprehensive evaluation, leading to the development of tailored therapeutic strategies. Multidisciplinary discussions foster a holistic understanding of the condition, facilitating personalized interventions geared towards optimal outcomes.

In essence, diagnosing dysphagia entails a diverse array of clinical assessments and specialized investigations, culminating in a thorough understanding of swallowing function and its complexities. By harnessing the expertise of diverse healthcare professionals, individuals grappling with swallowing difficulties receive comprehensive evaluations, paving the way for targeted interventions aimed at enhancing swallowing function and overall well-being.

Approaches to treating the condition

Dysphagia therapy is a comprehensive and multi-faceted endeavor, intricately tailored to address the individualized symptoms, severity, and medical history of each patient. The overarching goal is to enhance swallowing function and ultimately improve the quality of life for those affected. This multifaceted approach encompasses a range of treatment modalities, including various therapeutic techniques, dietary modifications, and, in rare cases, medical or surgical interventions.

Central to dysphagia therapy is the adjustment of food intake to align with the patient's swallowing capacity. This necessitates a tiered approach to dietary modifications, with different levels of food and drink consistency tailored to the severity of dysphagia. For individuals with severe dysphagia, initiation with a pureed or blended diet is typically recommended. As dysphagia severity lessens, progression to softer textures provided by the Level 2-Mechanical Soft Diet may be suitable. Moderate dysphagia may benefit from further modifications towards a more regular diet, facilitated by the Level 3 - Advanced or Soft Diet.

Integral to dysphagia treatment plans is the provision of targeted swallowing therapy administered by skilled speech-language pathologists. These professionals employ a variety of exercises aimed at strengthening relevant muscles, improving coordination, and enhancing overall swallowing function. Additionally, neuromuscular electrical stimulation (NMES) may be utilized to stimulate specific swallowing muscles in select cases.

In instances where dysphagia arises from underlying medical conditions, medication may be prescribed accordingly. For example, proton pump inhibitors are commonly used to alleviate esophageal irritation and inflammation associated with gastroesophageal reflux. Similarly, musculoskeletal abnormalities contributing to dysphagia may be addressed through interventions such as botulinum toxin injections.

In cases where structural abnormalities are identified as the root cause of dysphagia, surgical interventions may be considered. Procedures such as tumor removal, stricture dilation, or anatomical corrections aim to restore normal swallowing function and alleviate symptoms.

In extreme situations where dysphagia poses significant risks of dehydration and malnutrition, the insertion of a feeding tube may be warranted.

This ensures adequate nutrition and hydration by bypassing the oral phase of swallowing.

Behavioral strategies also play a crucial role in dysphagia management, focusing on techniques such as eating at a slower pace, taking smaller bites, and maintaining an upright posture during meals. Environmental modifications, including alterations in food presentation and texture, can further aid in swallowing efficiency.

Ultimately, dysphagia therapy is a dynamic and personalized process that evolves in response to the individual's changing needs and objectives over time. Regular monitoring and adjustment of the treatment plan are essential to optimize outcomes. Through a collaborative and interdisciplinary approach involving speech-language pathologists, dietitians, physicians, and other healthcare professionals, comprehensive care is delivered to enhance swallowing function and promote overall well-being in individuals with dysphagia.

CHAPTER V: LIVING WITH DYSPHAGIA: ADVICE AND PLANS

One crucial aspect of living with dysphagia involves dietary modifications tailored to meet specific requirements. This may entail altering the texture of meals through techniques such as pureeing or softening to facilitate easier swallowing. Collaborating closely with qualified professionals such as dietitians or speech-language pathologists is recommended to craft a personalized eating plan that addresses both swallowing issues and nutritional needs comprehensively.

In addition to dietary adjustments, cultivating mindful eating habits is paramount. Strategies such as consuming smaller portions, thoroughly chewing food, and maintaining an upright posture during meals can help simplify swallowing and reduce the risk of aspiration. Finding a quiet, distraction-free environment for meals can aid individuals with dysphagia in focusing on the chewing process, enhancing safety and comfort.

Hydration plays a crucial role in dysphagia management as well. Individuals are advised to maintain adequate hydration by sipping water in small quantities throughout the day rather than consuming large volumes at once, thus minimizing the risk of choking. Some individuals may benefit from thickening drinks to a more manageable consistency, as recommended by healthcare providers.

Regular physical activity is not only beneficial for overall health but can also contribute to dysphagia management. Specific exercises targeting and strengthening the muscles involved in swallowing may lead to improved swallowing function over time. Guidance from healthcare professionals, including physicians or speech therapists, is essential in designing and implementing an effective exercise regimen tailored to individual needs.

Social support plays a vital role in the journey of those living with dysphagia. Sharing the diagnosis with loved ones and caregivers enables them to provide better assistance and remain vigilant regarding necessary safety precautions. Recognizing symptoms of aspiration, such as coughing or difficulty breathing while eating, empowers loved ones to intervene promptly and mitigate potential consequences.

Furthermore, proactive scheduling of medical appointments is crucial for monitoring progress and making necessary adjustments to treatment plans. Regular consultations with healthcare experts, including specialists like speech-language pathologists, enable individuals to track improvements and address any emerging challenges promptly.

Effective management of dysphagia requires a holistic approach encompassing dietary modifications, mindful eating practices, hydration strategies, targeted exercises, social support, and proactive medical care. With the right support and interventions, individuals living with dysphagia can enhance their quality of life and effectively navigate the challenges associated with this condition, albeit requiring ongoing attention and care.

The responsibility of caregivers in managing dysphagia

Dysphagia, characterized by difficulty in swallowing, underscores the pivotal role of caregivers in navigating this complex disorder.

Caregivers undertake a multifaceted approach aimed at fostering safe and efficient swallowing as an integral aspect of daily patient care for those grappling with dysphagia.

Their responsibilities encompass a spectrum of interventions, ranging from ensuring optimal posture during meals to modifying food textures and consistencies to facilitate ease of swallowing. Vigilance regarding the manifestation of symptoms such as pain or aspiration necessitates meticulous monitoring of the patient's dietary intake, a task that caregivers undertake with unwavering diligence.

Collaboration with a diverse array of healthcare professionals, including nutritionists and speech-language pathologists, is indispensable in devising and implementing personalized strategies for the management and treatment of dysphagia. Through this interdisciplinary approach, caregivers gain access to a wealth of expertise and resources that are instrumental in optimizing patient outcomes.

Furthermore, caregivers extend invaluable emotional support and encouragement to individuals grappling with dysphagia, recognizing the profound impact this condition can have on an individual's overall quality of life. Their empathetic presence serves as a pillar of strength for patients navigating the challenges associated with dysphagia.

In order to discharge their duties effectively and ensure the holistic well-being of individuals with dysphagia, caregivers prioritize ongoing education and training in best practices, communication techniques, and procedural protocols. Equipped with comprehensive knowledge and skills, caregivers are empowered to navigate the complexities of dysphagia management with confidence and competence.

Ultimately, caregivers play an indispensable role in enhancing the health, safety, and quality of life of individuals affected by dysphagia, underscoring the profound impact of their unwavering dedication and compassionate care.

Avoiding Adverse Outcomes

In every domain, be it healthcare, project management, or daily routines, proactivity and meticulous planning stand as indispensable measures in preempting challenges and fostering smoother operations. Within the realm of healthcare, a comprehensive approach encompassing patient education, regular surveillance, and adherence to established protocols synergistically serves to mitigate the likelihood of complications. Emphasizing preventative interventions such as vaccinations, routine screenings, and lifestyle modifications is paramount for reducing the incidence of illnesses and adversities.

Effective communication between healthcare providers and patients is pivotal for ensuring a thorough understanding of illnesses and treatment regimens, thereby empowering individuals to actively participate in their healthcare journey. Furthermore, thorough risk assessment, continuous analysis, and periodic review constitute foundational elements in project management aimed at averting potential pitfalls. By identifying hazards early on, the development of mitigation strategies and contingency plans is streamlined, facilitating prompt and constructive resolution of challenges.

Fostering a culture of frequent communication among team members facilitates swift problem identification and resolution during project execution. Establishing realistic objectives, optimizing resource allocation, and maintaining adaptability are integral facets in circumventing obstacles and achieving project success. Likewise, in everyday life, individuals can preempt challenges by adopting proactive measures and prioritizing their health and well-being.

Strategies such as stress management, adequate rest, regular exercise, and balanced nutrition contribute to overall resilience and vitality. Effective time management, open communication, and proficient conflict resolution skills are instrumental in nurturing healthy relationships both in professional settings and personal spheres.

In essence, a proactive mindset, adherence to best practices, and adaptability are indispensable components in the realm of problem prevention. Whether it pertains to healthcare, project management, or daily routines, the fusion of knowledge, communication, and strategic foresight serves as the linchpin for minimizing risks and maximizing achievements.

CHAPTER VI: THE CONNECTION BETWEEN DIET AND DYSPHAGIA

The relationship between diet and the development of dysphagia, a medical condition characterized by difficulty swallowing, is profound and multifaceted. Food choices play a pivotal role in both the onset and progression of dysphagia, making the link between diet and the disorder intricate and nuanced. While certain foods and textures may exacerbate dysphagia symptoms, adopting a nutritious diet can significantly aid in managing swallowing difficulties.

Individuals afflicted with dysphagia often encounter challenges when consuming foods and beverages of varying textures. Swallowing difficulties can vary widely among affected individuals, with some experiencing issues with thick liquids while others struggle with solid foods. Consequently, modifying food texture becomes imperative to ensure safe and manageable swallowing. Healthcare professionals may recommend interventions such as thickened drinks, soft or pureed meals, or dietary adjustments aimed at minimizing sensory triggers.

Moreover, individuals with dysphagia must be vigilant about their dietary intake to prevent malnutrition and weight loss, which can result from reduced food consumption due to swallowing difficulties. Collaboratively, healthcare providers, including dietitians and speech-language pathologists, play a crucial role in ensuring that individuals with dysphagia receive adequate nutrition. This may involve implementing nutrient-rich diets and, in some cases, incorporating oral dietary supplements to address any nutritional deficiencies.

Conversely, certain dietary choices have the potential to exacerbate dysphagia symptoms or even contribute to its development. For instance, the consumption of acidic or spicy foods may irritate the esophagus, leading to inflammation and subsequent swallowing problems. Additionally, habits such as smoking and excessive alcohol consumption are associated with an increased risk of dysphagia and related conditions, such as esophageal cancer.

The management and treatment of dysphagia necessitate a comprehensive approach that encompasses dietary modifications tailored to address swallowing difficulties, maintenance of adequate nutrition, and avoidance of potential triggers. Healthcare providers serve as invaluable resources for individuals with dysphagia, offering guidance on optimal food choices and dietary strategies tailored to their specific condition and needs. Through collaborative efforts between patients and healthcare professionals, the impact of dysphagia on quality of life can be minimized, allowing individuals to effectively manage their condition and maintain overall well-being.

Comprehending Dysphagia and the Obstacles in Diet

Individuals grappling with dysphagia encounter significant challenges with swallowing, resulting in difficulties consuming both food and beverages. This condition can stem from a variety of sources, including neurological disorders, anatomical irregularities, or muscular dysfunction. As the ability to swallow becomes compromised, individuals with dysphagia often face profound dietary dilemmas.

A primary dietary concern for those with dysphagia is aspiration, wherein food or liquid mistakenly enters the airway instead of the esophagus, posing potential respiratory hazards. To mitigate this risk, dietary modifications, such as altering food consistency, may be imperative. This process involves adjusting the texture of meals and beverages to facilitate easier swallowing. Common adaptations include transitioning to pureed foods, thickened liquids, and modified textures achieved through mechanical alteration or softening techniques.

Moreover, individuals with dysphagia may grapple with inadequate food intake due to limitations on food options and textures, leading to concerns regarding malnutrition and dehydration. Addressing these nutritional needs while ensuring safe swallowing requires the expertise of healthcare professionals, including speech-language pathologists and dietitians, who can craft personalized meal plans tailored to individual requirements.

The psychological and social dimensions of dysphagia are equally significant to consider. Adjusting to altered eating habits and navigating dietary restrictions can evoke feelings of stress and isolation during mealtimes. Support from family members and caregivers plays a pivotal role in fostering a supportive and accommodating dining environment, thereby enhancing the overall dining experience and easing the burden for individuals with dysphagia.

Dysphagia represents a multifaceted challenge encompassing physiological, psychological, and social aspects. Implementing comprehensive strategies that encompass modifications to food consistency, nutritional support, and psychological well-being is essential in addressing the complex dietary issues associated with dysphagia. Effective management of dysphagia and enhancement of quality of life necessitate a collaborative approach involving healthcare providers, individuals affected by the condition, and their support networks.

The significance of adhering to a diet conducive to managing dysphagia

Individuals experiencing difficulty with swallowing should prioritize adopting a dysphagia-friendly dietary regimen tailored to their specific needs and challenges. This condition, often intertwined with various underlying health conditions such as neurological disorders, stroke, or aging, significantly impedes an individual's ability to consume food and beverages comfortably. By focusing on the textures of both solid foods and liquids, a dysphagia-friendly diet aims to mitigate the risks of choking and aspiration.

Beyond addressing immediate physical discomfort, the implementation of a dysphagia-friendly diet holds the potential to avert more severe complications in the future, such as malnutrition and dehydration. Healthcare professionals play a crucial role in enhancing the quality of life for individuals grappling with dysphagia by ensuring adequate intake of nourishing foods and facilitating enjoyable eating experiences through meal adaptations tailored to their unique requirements.

Furthermore, fostering social connections and maintaining interpersonal relationships constitute additional significant benefits of adhering to a dysphagia-friendly diet. Despite swallowing difficulties, individuals can still actively participate in the communal act of sharing meals with others through dietary modifications. This not only serves to alleviate emotional strain but also instills a sense of normalcy and inclusion, even amidst the challenges posed by a chronic illness.

Recognizing the multifaceted nature of dysphagia, a dysphagia-friendly diet emerges as an indispensable component of comprehensive healthcare. By addressing both the physical and emotional dimensions of this condition, it promotes a holistic and empathetic approach to patient care, affirming the importance of prioritizing the overall well-being and quality of life of individuals contending with swallowing difficulties.

Cooking Methods for Dysphagia Management

Addressing dysphagia often involves modifying the consistency and texture of food to facilitate safer and easier swallowing for individuals with this condition. One common technique is pureeing, which entails thoroughly processing or blending ingredients until they achieve a smooth, lump-free consistency. Additionally, softening food by mashing it with a fork or using a food processor is another method employed to aid in swallowing.

Another crucial aspect of dysphagia management is the thickening of liquids to reduce the risk of aspiration. Commercial thickeners such as starch or gum-based products are often added to liquids to increase viscosity. Incorporating sauces, gravies, or broths into dry dishes can also enhance moisture retention, making them easier to swallow.

For solid foods like vegetables and meats, various cooking methods such as boiling, steaming, or stewing can be utilized to soften their texture. It's important to chop or dice these foods into small, bite-sized pieces to minimize the risk of choking. Hard meats, raw vegetables, and fibrous fruits should be avoided to prevent further difficulty in swallowing.

Temperature is another consideration in managing dysphagia, as individuals may find it challenging or painful to swallow foods that are too hot or too cold. Providing foods at the preferred temperature of the individual can help alleviate discomfort during mealtime. Personalized adjustments tailored to individual preferences and needs play a pivotal role in dysphagia management.

Seeking guidance from professionals such as speech-language pathologists or nutritionists specialized in dysphagia management is highly recommended. These experts can offer tailored recommendations for food choices and cooking techniques based on the individual's specific condition. Gradually transitioning from softer to firmer textures through a process known as consistency gradation can also be beneficial in accommodating changes in swallowing ability over time.

A comprehensive approach to dysphagia treatment encompasses a variety of strategies tailored to the individual's needs. The safety and effectiveness of dietary modifications should be carefully evaluated in consultation with healthcare providers to ensure optimal outcomes for individuals with dysphagia.

CHAPTER VII: THE FUNDAMENTALS OF DYSPHAGIA DIETS

Individuals afflicted with dysphagia, a disorder characterized by the challenging of swallowing, are often prescribed meticulously crafted dietary regimens tailored to their unique needs. These dietary interventions aim to facilitate safe ingestion of food and beverages, mitigating the risks of choking or aspiration, wherein foreign substances infiltrate the airway, posing grave health hazards. The severity of the swallowing impairment dictates the extent of dietary modifications required, ranging from mild to severe restrictions.

Within the realm of dysphagia diets, several delineated levels cater to varying degrees of swallowing difficulty. These include the standard diet, chopped diet, minced and wet diet, and pureed diet. Individuals grappling with profound swallowing impediments may find solace in the pureed diet, where foods are meticulously blended to achieve a smooth, homogeneous consistency. Meanwhile, the minced and wet diet offers textures akin to finely chopped or minced foods, whereas the chopped diet permits consumption of small, bite-sized morsels. For individuals with milder swallowing challenges, adhering to the conventional diet with minor adaptations may suffice.

In crafting dysphagia diets, alterations in liquid consistency are as imperative as modifications in food textures. Thickening liquids to varying degrees, ranging from mildly thick to extremely thick, serves as a crucial strategy in averting aspiration incidents. Thickened liquids traverse the esophagus at a slower pace, reducing the likelihood of aspiration and enhancing safety during swallowing endeavors.

Careful consideration is also extended to the temperature of consumed meals and beverages, in addition to their texture and volume. Individuals grappling with swallowing difficulties often find extreme temperatures exacerbate their condition. Hence, it is advisable to serve both food and drinks at a moderate temperature to mitigate discomfort and optimize swallowing efficacy.

Collaborative efforts among healthcare professionals, including speech-language pathologists, dietitians, and caregivers, are indispensable in formulating individualized dietary plans for dysphagia patients. Regular assessments of swallowing function and nutritional status are paramount to ensure ongoing support for the individual's overall health and well-being. Through this multidisciplinary approach, tailored dietary interventions can be implemented to address the specific needs and challenges posed by dysphagia, fostering improved quality of life and nutritional adequacy for affected individuals.

An Examination of Dysphagia Dietary Classifications

The utilization of dysphagia diet levels offers individuals grappling with swallowing difficulties a systematic approach to managing their symptoms, thereby enhancing their capacity to consume food and beverages safely while mitigating the risk of aspiration. Typically recommended by medical professionals such as nutritionists or speech-language pathologists, these dietary regimens are tailored to the severity of swallowing impairment experienced by each individual.

A comprehensive breakdown of dysphagia diet levels typically encompasses the following tiers:

1. **Level 1: Pureed Diet**

   - Consistency: Food is meticulously blended to achieve a smooth, lump-free texture.

   - Examples: Pureed vegetables, fruits, meats, and grains.

   - Purpose: Suited for individuals with severe swallowing difficulties who necessitate minimal chewing and swallowing effort.

2. **Level 2: Mechanical Soft Diet**

   - Consistency: Foods possess a soft, moist texture and can be easily mashed with a fork.

   - Examples: Cooked or finely chopped fruits and vegetables, tender meats, and soft grains.

   - Purpose: Ideal for individuals with moderate swallowing challenges who can tolerate slightly textured foods.

3. **Level 3: Dysphagia Advanced**

   - Consistency: Foods resemble their natural state but are modified to facilitate easier swallowing.

   - Examples: Moist and well-cooked meats, soft fruits and vegetables, and finely chopped or ground foods.

   - Purpose: Geared towards individuals with mild to moderate dysphagia, offering increased variety in food options.

4. **Level 4: Regular Diet**

   - Consistency: Foods maintain their original textures without alteration.

   - Examples: Whole fruits and vegetables, meats of varying textures, and standard grains.

- Purpose: Recommended for individuals with minimal or no swallowing difficulties who can safely consume a regular diet without heightened risk of aspiration.

Importantly, the progression between dietary levels is contingent upon the individual's progress in swallowing therapy. Healthcare providers continuously assess and adjust diets based on the unique needs of each patient, facilitating a gradual and safe transition away from restrictive dietary regimens whenever feasible.

In the context of dysphagia, the risk of aspiration during fluid intake should be carefully managed across all diet levels. Thus, considerations such as adjusting food textures and utilizing thickened liquids should be incorporated into the dietary plan. Determining the appropriate thickness of thickened liquids is typically tailored to each individual's swallowing ability.

Individuals grappling with dysphagia are strongly advised to consult their healthcare providers before implementing any dietary modifications to ensure adequate nutrition and hydration while prioritizing safe eating practices. By adhering to personalized dietary recommendations, individuals can optimize their overall well-being while navigating the challenges associated with dysphagia effectively.

Different Phases of the Dysphagia Diet Levels and Recommended Recipes

LEVEL 1: PUREED DIET

Creamy Carrot Soup

Ingredients

2 cups cooked carrots

1 cup low-sodium chicken or vegetable broth

1/2 cup cooked rice or mashed sweet potatoes

Salt and pepper to taste

The Making

Blend all ingredients until smooth.

Heat and serve.

Nutritional Information

Calories 130

Protein 3g

Carbohydrates 28g

Fat 0.5g

Smooth Butternut Squash Soup

Ingredients

2 cups cooked butternut squash

1 cup low-sodium chicken or vegetable broth

1/2 cup cooked quinoa or mashed cauliflower

Salt and pepper to taste

The Making

Blend all ingredients until smooth.

Heat and serve.

Nutritional Information

Calories 140

Protein 4g

Carbohydrates 30g

Fat 1g

Silky Spinach Soup

Ingredients

2 cups cooked spinach

1 cup low-sodium chicken or vegetable broth

1/2 cup cooked white beans or mashed zucchini

Salt and pepper to taste

The Making

Blend all ingredients until smooth.

Heat and serve.

Nutritional Information

Calories 150

Protein 6g

Carbohydrates 27g

Fat 1g

Smooth Potato Leek Soup

Ingredients

2 cups cooked potatoes

1 cup low-sodium chicken or vegetable broth

1/2 cup cooked leeks (white part only)

Salt and pepper to taste

The Making

Blend all ingredients until smooth.

Heat and serve.

Nutritional Information

Calories 150

Protein 4g

Carbohydrates 30g

Fat 1g

Creamy Tomato Basil Soup

Ingredients

2 cups cooked tomatoes

1 cup low-sodium chicken or vegetable broth

1/2 cup cooked white beans or mashed carrots

Salt and pepper to taste

Fresh basil leaves for garnish (optional)

The Making

Blend all ingredients until smooth.

Heat and serve, garnishing with basil leaves if desired.

Nutritional Information

Calories 140

Protein 5g

Carbohydrates 27g

Fat 1g

Silky Mushroom Soup

Ingredients

2 cups cooked mushrooms

1 cup low-sodium chicken or vegetable broth

1/2 cup cooked barley or mashed parsnips

Salt and pepper to taste

The Making

Blend all ingredients until smooth.

Heat and serve.

Nutritional Information

Calories 145

Protein 6g

Carbohydrates 28g

Fat 1g

Creamy Asparagus Soup

Ingredients

2 cups cooked asparagus

1 cup low-sodium chicken or vegetable broth

1/2 cup cooked millet or mashed cauliflower

Salt and pepper to taste

The Making

Blend all ingredients until smooth.

Heat and serve.

Nutritional Information

Calories 135

Protein 5g

Carbohydrates 28g

Fat 1g

Velvety Red Pepper Soup

Ingredients

2 cups cooked red bell peppers

1 cup low-sodium chicken or vegetable broth

1/2 cup cooked lentils or mashed sweet potatoes

Salt and pepper to taste

The Making

Blend all ingredients until smooth.

Heat and serve.

 Nutritional Information

Calories 145

Protein 5g

Carbohydrates 29g

Fat 1g

Velvety Cauliflower Soup

Ingredients

2 cups cooked cauliflower

1 cup low-sodium chicken or vegetable broth

1/2 cup cooked oats or mashed turnips

Salt and pepper to taste

The Making

Blend all ingredients until smooth.

Heat and serve.

Nutritional Information

Calories 140

Protein 5g

Carbohydrates 29g

Fat 1.5g

Creamy Pea Soup

Ingredients

2 cups cooked peas

1 cup low-sodium chicken or vegetable broth

1/2 cup cooked brown rice or mashed pumpkin

Salt and pepper to taste

The Making

Blend all ingredients until smooth.

Heat and serve.

Nutritional Information

Calories 135

Protein 5g

Carbohydrates 28g

Fat 0.5g

Creamy Broccoli Soup:

Ingredients

2 cups steamed broccoli

1 cup low-sodium chicken or vegetable broth

1/2 cup cooked potatoes

Salt and pepper to taste

The Making

Blend all **Ingredients** until smooth.

Heat and serve.

Nutritional Information

Calories: 120

Protein: 5g

Carbohydrates: 25g

Fat: 1g

Mashed Sweet Potatoes with Cinnamon:

Ingredients

2 cups cooked sweet potatoes

1/4 cup unsweetened almond milk

1 teaspoon cinnamon

Pinch of salt

The Making

Blend sweet potatoes, almond milk, cinnamon, and salt until smooth.

Adjust consistency as needed.

Nutritional Information

Calories: 150

Protein: 2g

Carbohydrates: 35g

Fat: 1g

Pureed Turkey and Gravy:

Ingredients

1 cup cooked turkey

1/2 cup mashed potatoes

1/4 cup low-sodium turkey gravy

The Making

Blend turkey and mashed potatoes until smooth.

Add gravy and blend until well combined.

Nutritional Information

Calories: 220

Protein: 15g

Carbohydrates: 20g

Fat: 8g

Creamy Spinach and Ricotta:

Ingredients

2 cups cooked spinach

1/2 cup ricotta cheese

Nutmeg and salt to taste

The Making

Blend cooked spinach, ricotta, nutmeg, and salt until creamy.

Adjust thickness with water if needed.

Nutritional Information

Calories: 180

Protein: 10g

Carbohydrates: 8g

Fat: 12g

Pureed Chicken and Vegetable Casserole:

Ingredients

1 cup cooked chicken

1/2 cup cooked carrots

1/4 cup mashed potatoes

1/4 cup low-sodium chicken broth

The Making

Blend all **Ingredients** until smooth.

Add chicken broth for desired consistency.

Nutritional Information

Calories: 240

Protein: 20g

Carbohydrates: 15g

Fat: 10g

Creamy Avocado and Greek Yogurt Dip:

Ingredients

1 ripe avocado

1/2 cup plain Greek yogurt

Lemon juice, salt, and pepper to taste

The Making

Blend avocado, Greek yogurt, lemon juice, salt, and pepper until smooth.

Serve as a dip with soft crackers or pureed bread.

Nutritional Information

Calories: 200

Protein: 8g

Carbohydrates: 12g

Fat: 15g

Pureed Apple and Cinnamon Oatmeal:

Ingredients

1/2 cup cooked oats

1/2 cup unsweetened applesauce

1/4 teaspoon cinnamon

Water for desired consistency

The Making

Blend oats, applesauce, and cinnamon until smooth.

Adjust thickness with water.

Nutritional Information

Calories: 180

Protein: 4g

Carbohydrates: 40g

Fat: 2g

Pureed Pumpkin and Carrot Soup:

Ingredients

1 cup cooked pumpkin

1/2 cup cooked carrots

1/4 cup coconut milk

Curry powder, salt, and pepper to taste

The Making

Blend pumpkin, carrots, coconut milk, and spices until smooth.

Adjust thickness as desired.

Nutritional Information

Calories: 150

Protein: 2g

Carbohydrates: 25g

Fat: 6g

Pureed Blueberry and Banana Smoothie:

Ingredients

1/2 cup blueberries (fresh or frozen)

1 ripe banana

1/2 cup plain yogurt

Water for desired consistency

The Making

Blend blueberries, banana, and yogurt until smooth.

Add water to achieve the desired thickness.

Nutritional Information

Calories: 160

Protein: 5g

Carbohydrates: 35g

Fat: 2g

Creamy Cauliflower and Cheese Mash:

Ingredients

2 cups cooked cauliflower

1/4 cup grated cheddar cheese

1/4 cup unsweetened almond milk

Salt and pepper to taste

The Making

Blend cauliflower, cheddar cheese, almond milk, salt, and pepper until smooth.

Adjust consistency as needed.

Nutritional Information

Calories: 180

Protein: 8g

Carbohydrates: 15g

Fat: 10g

LEVEL 2: MECHANICAL SOFT DIET

Soft Vegetable and Quinoa Bowl:

Ingredients

1/2 cup cooked quinoa

1/2 cup soft-cooked mixed vegetables (zucchini, bell peppers, and carrots)

2 tablespoons olive oil

The Making

Combine cooked quinoa and vegetables, drizzle with olive oil.

Toss until well-mixed and serve.

Nutritional Information

Calories: 250

Protein: 7g

Carbohydrates: 30g

Fat: 12g

Soft Lentil and Vegetable Stew:

Ingredients

1/2 cup cooked lentils

1/2 cup soft-cooked vegetables (carrots, peas, and potatoes)

1/4 cup tomato sauce

The Making

Combine cooked lentils, soft vegetables, and tomato sauce.

Heat until warm and serve.

Nutritional Information

Calories: 200

Protein: 15g

Carbohydrates: 30g

Fat: 2g

Soft Turkey and Mashed Potatoes:

Ingredients

1 cup shredded cooked turkey

1/2 cup mashed potatoes

1/4 cup turkey gravy

The Making

Combine shredded turkey, mashed potatoes, and warm turkey gravy.

Mix until well-incorporated.

Nutritional Information

Calories: 250

Protein: 20g

Carbohydrates: 20g

Fat: 10g

Soft Vegetable and Chicken Stir-Fry:

Ingredients

1 cup soft-cooked mixed vegetables (carrots, peas, and green beans)

1/2 cup shredded cooked chicken

2 tablespoons low-sodium soy sauce

The Making

Stir-fry vegetables until soft, then add shredded chicken and soy sauce.

Cook until well-blended and serve.

Nutritional Information

Calories: 180

Protein: 15g

Carbohydrates: 15g

Fat: 7g

Mashed Avocado and Tuna Salad:

Ingredients

1/2 ripe avocado, mashed

1/2 cup canned tuna, drained

1 tablespoon mayonnaise

The Making

Combine mashed avocado, tuna, and mayonnaise.

Mix until well-blended and serve.

Nutritional Information

Calories: 220

Protein: 15g

Carbohydrates: 10g

Fat: 15g

Tender Chicken and Rice Casserole

Ingredients

1 cup shredded cooked chicken

1/2 cup cooked white rice

1/4 cup chicken broth

1/4 cup grated cheese (optional)

The Making

Mix shredded chicken, cooked rice, and chicken broth in a baking dish.

Sprinkle grated cheese on top if desired.

Bake at 350°F (175°C) for 20-25 minutes until heated through and cheese is melted.

Serve warm.

Nutritional Information

Calories 280

Protein 22g

Carbohydrates 25g

Fat 9g

Tender Beef and Vegetable Stew

Ingredients

1 cup cooked beef, diced

1/2 cup cooked carrots, diced

1/4 cup cooked peas

1/4 cup beef broth

Salt and pepper to taste

The Making

Combine cooked beef, carrots, peas, and beef broth in a pot.

Season with salt and pepper to taste.

Simmer over low heat for 15-20 minutes until heated through.

Serve hot.

Nutritional Information

Calories 260

Protein 18g

Carbohydrates 15g

Fat 12g

Creamy Chicken and Vegetable Pasta

Ingredients

1 cup shredded cooked chicken

1/2 cup cooked pasta

1/4 cup cooked mixed vegetables (carrots, peas, broccoli)

1/4 cup low-sodium chicken broth

2 tablespoons plain Greek yogurt

The Making

Combine shredded chicken, cooked pasta, mixed vegetables, and chicken broth in a saucepan.

Stir in Greek yogurt until well-incorporated.

Heat gently over low heat until warmed through.

Serve hot.

Nutritional Information

Calories 270

Protein 20g

Carbohydrates 25g

Fat 10g

Soft Beef and Potato Casserole

Ingredients

1 cup cooked ground beef

1/2 cup mashed potatoes

1/4 cup beef gravy

1/4 cup cooked green beans

Salt and pepper to taste

The Making

Layer cooked ground beef, mashed potatoes, and green beans in a baking dish.

Pour beef gravy evenly over the top.

Bake at 350°F (175°C) for 20-25 minutes until heated through.

Serve warm.

Nutritional Information

Calories 280

Protein 18g

Carbohydrates 20g

Fat 12g

Smooth Turkey and Lentil Soup

Ingredients

1 cup shredded cooked turkey

1/2 cup cooked lentils

1/4 cup low-sodium chicken broth

1/4 cup diced tomatoes (canned or fresh)

1/2 teaspoon dried herbs (such as thyme or rosemary)

The Making

Combine shredded turkey, cooked lentils, chicken broth, diced tomatoes, and dried herbs in a pot.

Simmer over low heat for 15-20 minutes until heated through and flavors meld.

Serve hot.

Nutritional Information

Calories 260

Protein 20g

Carbohydrates 20g

Fat 9g

Mild Fish and Vegetable Bake

Ingredients

1 cup cooked white fish, flaked

1/2 cup cooked mashed potatoes

1/4 cup cooked carrots, diced

1/4 cup low-sodium fish or vegetable broth

Lemon zest for garnish

The Making

Layer cooked fish, mashed potatoes, and diced carrots in a baking dish.

Pour fish or vegetable broth over the top.

Bake at 375°F (190°C) for 20-25 minutes until heated through.

Garnish with lemon zest before serving.

Nutritional Information

Calories 270

Protein 20g

Carbohydrates 20g

Fat 10g

Creamy Vegetable and Bean Casserole

Ingredients

1 cup cooked mixed vegetables (carrots, peas, corn)

1/2 cup cooked white beans

1/4 cup low-sodium vegetable broth

1/4 cup shredded cheese (optional)

Salt and pepper to taste

The Making

Combine mixed vegetables, white beans, and vegetable broth in a baking dish.

Sprinkle shredded cheese on top if desired.

Bake at 350°F (175°C) for 20-25 minutes until heated through and cheese is melted.

Serve warm.

Nutritional Information

Calories 250

Protein 15g

Carbohydrates 30g

Fat 8g

Soft Salmon and Quinoa Salad

Ingredients

1 cup cooked salmon, flaked

1/2 cup cooked quinoa

1/4 cup Greek yogurt

1 tablespoon lemon juice

Salt and pepper to taste

The Making

Mix cooked salmon, quinoa, Greek yogurt, and lemon juice in a bowl.

Season with salt and pepper to taste.

Chill in the refrigerator for 30 minutes before serving.

Serve cold.

Nutritional Information

Calories 270

Protein 23g

Carbohydrates 20g

Fat 10g

Gentle Tuna and Pasta Bake

Ingredients

1 cup cooked pasta

1/2 cup canned tuna, drained

1/4 cup creamy Alfredo sauce

1/4 cup frozen peas, thawed

The Making

Combine cooked pasta, tuna, Alfredo sauce, and peas in a baking dish.

Mix until well-combined.

Bake at 375°F (190°C) for 20-25 minutes until bubbly and heated through.

Serve warm.

Nutritional Information

Calories 290

Protein 22g

Carbohydrates 25g

Fat 11g

Tender Turkey and Vegetable Soup

Ingredients

1 cup shredded cooked turkey

1/2 cup cooked mixed vegetables (carrots, peas, corn)

1/4 cup low-sodium chicken broth

Salt and pepper to taste

The Making

Combine shredded turkey, mixed vegetables, and chicken broth in a pot.

Season with salt and pepper to taste.

Simmer over low heat for 15-20 minutes until vegetables are tender and flavors meld.

Serve hot.

Nutritional Information

Calories 250

Protein 20g

Carbohydrates 15g

Fat 10g

Soft Spinach and Feta Omelette:

Ingredients

2 eggs, beaten

1/2 cup cooked spinach

2 tablespoons crumbled feta cheese

The Making

Cook beaten eggs in a non-stick pan, add cooked spinach, and sprinkle feta on top.

Fold the omelette and cook until the cheese is melted.

Nutritional Information

Calories: 220

Protein: 15g

Carbohydrates: 5g

Fat: 15g

Soft Baked Salmon with Lemon Dill Sauce:

Ingredients

1 cup baked or poached salmon, flaked

2 tablespoons Greek yogurt

1 tablespoon fresh dill, chopped

Lemon juice to taste

The Making

Mix flaked salmon with Greek yogurt, dill, and lemon juice.

Warm before serving.

Nutritional Information

Calories: 230

Protein: 20g

Carbohydrates: 3g

Fat: 15g

Soft Chicken and Cheese Quesadilla:

Ingredients

1 small soft tortilla

1/2 cup shredded cooked chicken

1/4 cup shredded cheese

The Making

Place shredded chicken and cheese on one half of the tortilla.

Fold the tortilla and warm until the cheese is melted.

Nutritional Information

Calories: 280

Protein: 20g

Carbohydrates: 20g

Fat: 14g

Soft Apple and Cinnamon Oatmeal:

Ingredients

1/2 cup cooked oats

1/2 cup soft-cooked apples

1/4 teaspoon cinnamon

Water for desired consistency

The Making

Combine cooked oats, soft apples, and cinnamon.

Adjust thickness with water if needed.

Nutritional Information

Calories: 200

Protein: 4g

Carbohydrates: 40g

Fat: 2g

Soft Banana and Peanut Butter Smoothie:

Ingredients

1 ripe banana

2 tablespoons smooth peanut butter

1/2 cup plain yogurt

Water for desired consistency

The Making

Blend banana, peanut butter, and yogurt until smooth.

Add water to achieve the desired thickness.

Nutritional Information

Calories: 280

Protein: 8g

Carbohydrates: 30g

Fat: 16g

LEVEL 3: ADVANCED OR SOFT DIET

Grilled Chicken and Quinoa Salad:

Ingredients

1 cup grilled chicken breast, diced

1/2 cup cooked quinoa

Mixed salad greens

Olive oil and balsamic vinegar for dressing

The Making

Toss diced grilled chicken and cooked quinoa with mixed salad greens.

Drizzle with olive oil and balsamic vinegar for dressing.

Nutritional Information

Calories: 300

Protein: 25g

Carbohydrates: 20g

Fat: 12g

Shrimp and Vegetable Stir-Fry:

Ingredients

1/2 cup cooked shrimp, peeled and deveined

1 cup stir-fried mixed vegetables (broccoli, bell peppers, and snap peas)

1 tablespoon low-sodium soy sauce

The Making

Stir-fry shrimp and mixed vegetables with soy sauce until cooked.

Serve over rice or noodles.

Nutritional Information

Calories: 250

Protein: 20g

Carbohydrates: 15g

Fat: 10g

Soft Lentil and Spinach Curry:

Ingredients

1/2 cup cooked lentils

1 cup cooked spinach

1/4 cup coconut milk

Curry powder, salt, and pepper to taste

The Making

Combine cooked lentils and spinach with coconut milk and spices.

Simmer until heated through and serve over rice.

Nutritional Information

Calories: 280

Protein: 15g

Carbohydrates: 35g

Fat: 10g

Soft Beef and Mushroom Stroganoff:

Ingredients

1/2 cup cooked beef strips

1/2 cup sautéed mushrooms

2 tablespoons sour cream

Egg noodles or rice for serving

The Making

Mix cooked beef and sautéed mushrooms with

sour cream.

Serve over egg noodles or rice.

Nutritional Information

Calories: 320

Protein: 25g

Carbohydrates: 15g

Fat: 18g

Soft Salmon and Asparagus Risotto:

Ingredients

1/2 cup baked or grilled salmon, flaked

1/2 cup cooked asparagus

1/2 cup risotto

Parmesan cheese for garnish

The Making

Combine flaked salmon, cooked asparagus, and risotto.

Garnish with Parmesan cheese before serving.

Nutritional Information

Calories: 320

Protein: 20g

Carbohydrates: 25g

Fat: 15g

Soft Spinach and Feta Stuffed Chicken Breast:

Ingredients

2 boneless, skinless chicken breasts

1 cup cooked spinach

2 tablespoons crumbled feta cheese

The Making

Butterfly chicken breasts and stuff with cooked spinach and feta.

Bake until chicken is cooked through.

Nutritional Information

Calories: 280

Protein: 35g

Carbohydrates: 5g

Fat: 12g

Soft Egg Salad Sandwich:

Ingredients

2 boiled eggs, mashed

2 tablespoons mayonnaise

Lettuce leaves

Soft bread or roll

The Making

Mix mashed boiled eggs with mayonnaise.

Spread the egg salad on soft bread or a roll, and add lettuce.

Nutritional Information

Calories: 250

Protein: 15g

Carbohydrates: 20g

Fat: 15g

Soft Tofu and Vegetable Stir-Fry:

Ingredients

1/2 cup soft tofu, cubed

1 cup stir-fried mixed vegetables (broccoli, carrots, and bell peppers)

1 tablespoon teriyaki sauce

The Making

Stir-fry soft tofu and mixed vegetables with teriyaki sauce until heated.

Serve over rice or noodles.

Nutritional Information

Calories: 230

Protein: 15g

Carbohydrates: 20g

Fat: 10g

Soft Turkey and Cranberry Wrap:

Ingredients

1/2 cup shredded cooked turkey

2 tablespoons cranberry sauce

Soft tortilla or wrap

Lettuce for added texture

The Making

Mix shredded turkey with cranberry sauce.

Spread the mixture on a soft tortilla, add lettuce, and wrap.

Nutritional Information

Calories: 280

Protein: 20g

Carbohydrates: 30g

Fat: 10g

Soft Mango and Banana Smoothie Bowl:

Ingredients

1 ripe mango, peeled and diced

1 ripe banana

1/2 cup plain yogurt

Toppings: granola, sliced almonds, or chia seeds

The Making

Blend mango, banana, and yogurt until smooth.

Pour into a bowl and top with granola, sliced almonds, or chia seeds.

Nutritional Information

Calories: 280

Protein: 8g

Carbohydrates: 50g

Fat: 6g

CHAPTER VIII: LASTLY!

In concluding our exploration of dysphagia within the confines of this book, it becomes increasingly evident that this condition extends far beyond a mere impediment to swallowing. Rather, it represents a multifaceted challenge that permeates various aspects of an individual's life, profoundly impacting their physical health, emotional well-being, and overall quality of life. Throughout our journey, we've delved into the intricate nuances of dysphagia, dissecting its myriad causes, manifestations, diagnostic approaches, and treatment modalities.

Yet, amidst the intricacies and challenges, there exists a beacon of hope—a testament to the resilience of the human spirit and the remarkable strides made in the field of dysphagia management. Through interdisciplinary collaboration, innovative interventions, and a steadfast commitment to patient-centered care, individuals grappling with dysphagia can find solace in the prospect of improved swallowing function and enhanced quality of life.

Moreover, our exploration has underscored the critical importance of raising awareness and fostering understanding of dysphagia among healthcare professionals, caregivers, and the broader community. By dispelling misconceptions, reducing stigma, and advocating for greater access to comprehensive dysphagia care, we can create a more supportive and inclusive environment for those affected by this condition.

Looking toward the future, the landscape of dysphagia management holds promise for continued progress and innovation. With ongoing research, technological advancements, and a commitment to evidence-based practice, we can further refine our understanding of dysphagia and develop more effective strategies for its prevention, diagnosis, and treatment.

However, it's essential to acknowledge that the journey through dysphagia is not without its challenges. Individuals living with dysphagia, along with their caregivers and healthcare providers, must navigate a complex and often daunting path filled with uncertainty and setbacks. Yet, it is within these moments of adversity that the true strength of the human spirit shines brightest, as individuals demonstrate remarkable resilience, courage, and determination in the face of adversity.

As we close this chapter on dysphagia, let us carry forward the lessons learned, the insights gained, and the unwavering commitment to improving the lives of those affected by this condition. Let us continue to advocate for greater awareness, foster empathy and understanding, and work tirelessly toward a future where dysphagia no longer serves as a barrier to living a full and meaningful life.

Together, we can pave the way toward a brighter tomorrow, where individuals with dysphagia can thrive, flourish, and reclaim their rightful place in the world.